FITNESS
is a
Feeling

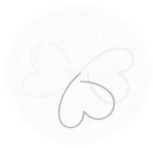

Heather Roselle

ISBN 978-1-7388693-0-5

Dedicated to the YFC Tribe.

Our conversations over the last ten years
have inspired this collection.

Thank you wise women!

Books change the lives
of readers who read them.

Books also change the lives
of authors who write them.

CHANDLER BOLT

Contents

Be around
the light bringers,
the magic makers,
the world shifters,
the game shakers.
They challenge, uplift
and expand you.
These heartbeats are
your people.
These people are
your tribe.

UNKNOWN

For

The woman who has yet to experience the joys of feeling fit.

As in never.

This same woman knows the value of fitness as it relates to personal wellness, yet the habit remains elusive.

> She thinks about it.
>
> Reads about it.
>
> Watches videos about it.
>
> Talks about it.

Still, the information or inspirations observed have yet to transfer consistently into her life.

There are literally millions of humans, experts and laypersons alike, offering advice on how to get fit.

This is my contribution, in the hopes the woman I have in mind begins her journey to feeling fit.

> Feeling fit for the rest of her life!

From

A quieter side of fitness, infused with a lifetime of conversations.

Every morsel of wisdom included in this book has been generated by conversations with real women.

Women who might hold celebrity status with their children or grandchildren or family or friends, but their images and their stories are not viewed or liked by millions of followers.

This is not a collection of get fit promises or guarantees or shortcuts or promotions.

This is a series of invitations for you to step onto a clear fitness path designed by you for your life.

One day at a time:

> A bit of reading.
>
> A bit of reflecting.
>
> A bit of moving.
>
> A bit of inspiration.

Welcome to your journey!

Pronouns

I identify with the pronouns she/her.

My book is written from this perspective, but it is not meant to exclude others with an alternate identity.

If the content within this book speaks to you, feel free to substitute your pronouns and take this journey with us.

Discovering fitness is personal and at the same time universally inclusive when YOU become the journey.

Life is best lived by
focusing on
your aspirations
and dancing through
all other distractions.

YOGI TEA AFFIRMATION

But Wait

Where are all the pictures...

Of the author?

Of the exercises?

If you've flipped through the book, you have noticed there are no pictures of me or anyone else doing the exercises.

The majority of fitness books have photos or video links demonstrating the author or models doing the exercises while living their best life.

This fitness book has words plus spaces and places for you to think, move and feel without pictures, images or photos.

By design.

On a sensory level, the design intentionally decreases what you see to increase your awareness of how you feel.

When you begin to feel fit, you will see everything from a different lens.

*I'm not a
healing guru...
I'm just a
curious cat.*

CHARLOTTE CHURCH

Conceptualize

It doesn't matter where
you start,
you need to
start somewhere.

KELLY STARRETT

You Are Here

It's essential to understand and continually reset your personal GPS:

Global Positioning Sensor.

This unique sensor encompasses your experiences, your strengths and your environment.

It indicates where you've been, where you are and positions you for the future.

Because our minds are often full, optimization of your GPS creates space to think mindfully.

This simplification allows you to focus on practicing fitness, rather than perfecting being fit.

Isn't life a series of practices with fleeting moments of near perfection?

Think about it...

This will be a journey worth documenting.

Not in a fitness log kind of way; in a way that allows you to be present, to look back and to consider the future.

Not his-story per se, her-story...YOUR-story!

I encourage you to select a method of capturing what you did, when you did it and how it felt.

What format appeals to you the most:

    Paper, scrapbook, journal?

    Tablet, voice recording, photography?

    Something else?

How do you create solutions to problems?

    Talking?

    Writing?

    Something else?

Where is a space that facilitates thinking clearly?

    Is it accessible anytime, any day?

Beginning

Go to a place where you think best.

What method of documentation did you select:

> Is it simple?
>
> Can you access it with or without WiFi?

Mindset

A mantra is a positive word or a phrase you repeat over and over to help develop focus.

Create a phrase, 5 words or less, to welcome yourself to this journey.

Some examples:

> 5 words - No time like the present.
>
> 4 words - And so it begins.
>
> 3 words - I am ready.
>
> 2 words - Sun's out.
>
> 1 word - Amplify.

Closing

If you haven't done so already, record today's date.

The journey of daily practice has begun!

When asked why,
at the age of 93,
did legendary cellist
Pablo Casals practice
three hours a day?

His response:
I'm beginning to
notice some
improvement.

PABLO CASALS

Your Map

Keep in mind this book is like a roadmap with you in the driver's seat.

Rather than prescribing a route for you to follow, simply begin without expectations, limitations or timelines.

This map invites you to be open, curious and patient.

The process invites you to interact with a few pages a day — slowing down the flow of information to deepen your connection with the creative process of practicing fitness every day.

While I have collated the chapters in the sequence that follows, you are free to navigate them in any order that works for you.

> Take detours when you need to.
>
> Stay a bit longer when you want to.
>
> Exceed the speed limit if you decide to.

Energy patterns...

Think about the rhythm of your days and weeks:

What commitments are predictable?

What elements fluctuate?

Is there a time or a day or a space where you notice:

Your energy is consistently higher than other times, days or spaces?

Your energy is consistently lower than other times, days or spaces?

How is your energy connected to:

Sleep?

Nutrition?

Hydration?

Stress?

How do you *recharge* when your energy is low?

Beginning	Return to that place where you think best. At a time of the day when you feel most energetic. Smile. Just to yourself, for yourself.
Mindset	When you think about this fitness roadmap: 　What are you most curious to discover? 　What are you most determined to avoid?
Closing	Smile again.

Continue...

*A journey of
one thousand miles
begins with
a single step.*

LAO TZU

Start by Stopping

All too often the decision to be fit, to become fit or to make more time for fitness results in radical lifestyle changes:

>Too early!

>Too intense!

>Too much movement!

>Too little to eat!

>Too impossible to sustain!

It took a period of time and a catalogue of life experiences to arrive here.

Instead of revolutionizing your life in a nanosecond, let's use your wisdom to make small, day-to-day changes for the rest of your life.

Trust...

>Fitness isn't a destination.

>Feeling fit is a journey.

>You are the navigator.

Your revolutions...

It seems humans are willing to try almost anything to improve their overall health or appearance.

There may even be some entertaining experiments and purchases in your past.

Some of you may remember the cabbage soup diet or the weight loss magic of sauna suits.

Or the temptation to purchase a Thigh Master or invest in a library of Jane Fonda VHS tapes.

With a sense of humor, take some time to recall some of those lifestyle or fitness fads or trends you have tried — try framing these memories in the context of plus, minus and interesting!

What did you try?		
Plus	Minus	Interesting

Beginning

Return to that place where you think best.

Or, try a new space.

Pause all connections to create a short DND:
Do Not Disturb.

» Silence your phone, email, messages, media or any other notifications.

Mindset

Take a moment to consider this question:

» What is a logical, simple, inexpensive lifestyle change you could make at this moment in time?

Record your considerations.

Now, commit to making this logical, simple, inexpensive lifestyle change happen within the next 48 hours.

Closing

Reconnect.

Carry on with your day.

Think.
Feel.
Be.

Don't you know
they're talkin' about
a revolution...
it sounds like
a whisper.

TRACY CHAPMAN

Deception

The act of starting is sometimes disguised as the art of delaying.

> Or stalling.

> Or procrastinating.

You might be familiar with this pattern.

You have a goal, something you want to change or achieve, but before you officially begin, you focus on what you think you need to get started.

This process is exciting, the focal point is a concept or an idea as opposed to taking steps towards a change.

By the time the items or systems are purchased or organized, your enthusiastic spark fizzles to the point it seems easier to abandon your goal and continue along a familiar path, unchanged — other than, perhaps, a growing, deep-rooted disappointment.

This journey to fitness begins where you are.

> With what you already have!

You know...

Everyone has experience with procrastination; otherwise known as the fine art of putting off what needs to be done.

   If you are like most people, you have your own style.

Make a short, honest list of your go to avoidance this & that strategies:

When I avoid doing that...

I distract myself with this...

🖤

Beginning

Go to today's reserved fitness space.

Pause all connections to create DND.

Sit or stand, aware of your posture, with your eyes open or closed:

> Notice what happens when you inhale.
> Notice what happens when you exhale.

Now, take 6 breaths.

Longer, deeper, more relaxing than how you usually breathe.

Mindset

Open your eyes and record one positive, powerful, motivational word to set the tone for the rest of your day.

> If more words come to mind, record them all and then select one.

Repeat it, out loud or silently to yourself.

Closing

Reconnect and continue with your day as planned.

Re-fueled with your own motivational word!

*Procrastination is
like a credit card –
it's a lot of fun
until you get the bill!*

CHRISTOPHER PARKE

Why Now

Collective wisdom perpetually highlights the positive connection between personal fitness and individual health.

The simple, universal and consistent message is:

> A fit body is better able to deal with infections, disease and stress.

And yet, the habit of fitness remains elusive for many.

This marks an important place to pause.

A space for you to state your purpose.

Your voice...

Your decisions.

    Your life.

Not the medical experts.

    Not your internal critic.

Just your authentic self.

    At this point in time.

Without pausing to think, edit or judge, make a list of reasons why YOU want to prioritize your personal fitness at this point in your life.

Your reasons why now...

Beginning

Relocate to your fitness space.

Establish DND.

Sit or stand with increased awareness:

> Where are your feet?
>
> Can you lengthen your spine to feel comfortably taller?
>
> Are your arms relaxed by your side?

Breath Awareness: eyes open or closed.

> Place one hand on your navel.
>
> Invite the belly to inflate when you breathe in; direct the belly to deflate as you breathe out.

Take 6 more belly breaths, exploring longer inhales and exhales.

Mindset

With your breath-infused mind, reread your answers to why now?

Take 3 more breaths.

Closing

End your DND.

Carry on with your day .

With a greater sense
of knowing why!

What you think,
you become.
What you feel,
you attract.
What you imagine,
you create.

BUDDHA

Censorship

Words can be heard, spoken, written, seen, thought and read.

They are powerful.

They inspire action.

They influence energy.

They shape emotions.

Although often synonymous with all things fitness, for the time being, the following words are censored:

~~Cardio~~

~~Conditioning~~

~~Calories~~

~~Competition~~

~~Carbs~~

~~Comparison~~

Your words shape your actions, energy and emotions.

So, let's refine your fitness language.

Your narrative...

The words you think, say and dream become:

Your past, present and future.

Have a quick look back at your her-story to take note of your fitness words...

Then, define your fitness is a feeling language by considering:

What words do YOU want included?

What words do YOU want excluded?

Beginning

Relocate to your fitness space and disconnect.

Sit or stand with postural, spine and foot awareness.

Breath Awareness: eyes open or closed.

> When you breathe in, lift your arms in any direction.
> When you breathe out, lower your arms.

Feel your breath start and end at your navel center — notice where your breath travels.

Repeat this breath and arm movement 5-7 more times.

Mindset

Your words are powerful.

This is your narrative.

Closing

Reconnect and carry on.

*The human body is extraordinary...
so are you!*

A strong woman knows
she has strength enough
for the journey.

A woman of strength
knows it is in the
journey where she will
become strong.

Anonymous

Overexposed

There is no shortage of fitness-related images, articles or footage. Within moments, at any point in the day, you are reminded that fitness is for:

Young or old.

Oversized or undersized.

Athletes or non-athletes.

The end result is image-exposure fatigue:

You could look like that!

You should be doing this!

You need to purchase this to do that so you can be a better person than you are right now!

Readers, viewers, followers and subscribers are skimming the surfaces of how to get fit.

Watching and listening, but not moving!

So many ideas.

So many suggestions.

Still, so little movement.

Your exposure...

Do you follow a wellness personality or seek sites for fitness inspiration?

Guesstimate:

How much time do you spend finding, following or fetching on social media?

Quick analysis:

Is the content entertaining or informative?

Now, select 1-3 personalities and dig a bit deeper:

Who...

What is their expertise or claim to fame?

What have you watched or read then added to your life?

Would you categorize the content to be entertaining, informative or something else?

Fitness Practice ♡ Practice Fitness

Beginning

Relocate to your fitness space.

Turn all screens off.

Notifications silenced. Music is optional.

Sit or stand with foot, spine and body awareness.

Breath Awareness:

When you breathe in, open your eyes and lift your arms in any direction.

When you breathe out, close your eyes and lower your arms.

Repeat this breath and arm movement 5 more times.

Movement

If you are standing, take a seat.

If you are sitting, stand on your feet.

Repeat this sit-stand transition 3-5 more times.

Mindset

Now close your eyes and take 3 breaths.

Savor your emerging expertise.

Closing

Reconnect and continue with your day as planned!

You,
your body,
your movements,
your expertise!

Changing our habits can be hard at first, messy in the middle, and gorgeous at the end.

ROBIN SHARMA

A Fresh Take

The wellness industry has a long history and, so it seems, an endless future as the struggle for humans to be well in body, mind and spirit becomes more complex, more elusive and, by times, more depressing.

You have more access to information and instruction today than at any other time in history.

Yet, health or wellness statistics in many countries indicate increasing numbers of humans are diagnosed with chronic disease, categorized as obese, die of stroke, manage arthritis and/or monitor varying degrees of diabetes.

While genetics may play a role in these poor health statistics, lifestyle remains a key element in diminishing or augmenting *dis-ease*.

As such, you will find an abundance of diet, exercise and psychology advice from experts and celebrities alike.

Many of these offerings might work for some, but you have not found the right fit for you.

So, take a break from health stats and editorials — let's highlight some of your current strengths.

Your exposure...

Think about you for a moment.

Specifically, your ability to move. Open your mind to consider the regular things you do in a typical day:

> Things like lifting toddlers, walking to and from transit stops, cleaning your own house, taking a weekly dance class, gardening, riding a bicycle...

Now...make a list of typical ways you move every day:

Think about you for another moment.

Specifically, what you think being healthy generally looks like or feels like:

> Things like good sleep habits; love eating green vegetables; having healthy hair, skin, nails, teeth...

Now...make a list of your wellness indicators:

Simply, finish the phrases:

I move best when...

The healthiest part of me is...

Beginning

Move into your fitness space.

Customize the elements based on your energy indicators:

> Light?
> Sound?
> Devices?

Breath Awareness:
> Sit or stand.
> Eyes open or closed.
> Arms still or in motion.

When you breathe in, finish this sentence:
> I am...

When you breathe out, finish this sentence:
> I am...

Mindset

Smile.

Acknowledge this moment.

Another completed fitness practice.

Closing

Reconnect and carry on with your day.

*Your smile is like the sun
shining on the center
of who you are,
highlighting your strengths.*

*Your body is a
self-sustaining
work of brilliance.*

JILL MILLER

Another Take

Trending media images of fitness are simply redundant.

Bodies, of all shapes and sizes, are captured, usually wearing various brands of form-fitting apparel, on location, be that outdoors or indoors, doing something related to fitness.

Yet, fitness is not exclusively defined by body weight, clothing size or a reflection in the mirror.

Fitness is much more than what we see, weigh or measure.

When achieved, it's more like a state of being.

Comfortable in your own skin.

Confident stepping into life's challenges and celebrations.

Strong enough to do what matters most every day.

Your take...

Can you recall a time in your life when you felt:

    Comfortable.

    Confident.

    Strong enough to do what mattered most!

When did you feel this way...

Where were you...

How did it feel...

It will be interesting to gaze, momentarily, towards your future self:

Can you predict how your fitness might feel in the future?

Beginning

Move into your space.

» Disconnect from distractions.

» Reconnect with your feet, legs, spine and arms.

Breath Work: select a number of breaths for your breath work:

» Eyes open or closed.

» Arms still or in motion.

Movement

Your Legs:
Begin seated.
Inhale when you stand up.
Exhale when you sit back down.

» Is this a day to sit-stand from a different seat: lower, less stable, different?

» Repeat stand-sit 4-6 more times.

Your Arms:
Begin standing.
Place your hands on a desk, a wall, a counter or a sturdy table.

» Allow your arms to bear the weight of your body with your feet on the floor.

» Simply bend your elbows as much as comfortable, then straighten.

» Repeat 2 more times.

Closing

Step back into your day.

One day at a time;
a bit stronger each day.

Few people actually want to be fit.

Most just want to look fit.

Erwan Le Corre

Fitness is

Beneficial for...

    Sleeping well.

    Eating well.

    Moving well.

    Living well.

Possible for...

    All ages.

    All athletic backgrounds.

    All body types.

    All budgets.

Also...

    Energizing.

    Stress releasing.

    Life enhancing.

Close yet remote...

If fitness is so readily accessible and so beneficial, what has prevented you from creating the right fitness formula for you?

Again, non-judgmentally, take a moment to consider some of your obstacles:

Identify the permanent barriers you live with:

Identify the barriers you can navigate around:

What if you discovered a way to navigate over, under, around or through these barriers:

How might your overall wellbeing change:

Beginning

Move into your practice space.

Set your devices. Set your body. Set your mind.

Breath Work: decide on the number of breaths.

» Eyes open or closed.
» Seated or standing.
» Arms still or in motion.

Movement

Your Legs:

» Inhale to stand, exhale to sit.
» Complete 6-8 sit-stand repetitions.

Your Arms:

» Place your hands on a desk, a wall, a counter or a sturdy table.
» Complete 2-4 push-up repetitions.

Air Sharpie:

Picture the shape of a circle.

Imagine there is a sharpie on the center of your chin...

» Slowly draw a circle in one direction, then the other.

Imagine that same sharpie on your right elbow...

» Slowly draw 2 circles in different directions.
» Repeat with your left elbow.

Repeat with your heels...

» One at a time. Slowly.

Mindset

Refocus your mind for your breath work:

    Eyes open or closed.

    Seated or standing.

    Arms still or in motion.

Sometimes the practice is the same.

Sometimes it changes.

Your daily habit of practicing fitness remains consistent.

Closing

Reconnect with your day.

Fitness is something
you practice
every day.

Reflection

When you look at the journey thus far, have you noticed a pattern of consistency — spaces that work well for you and your fitness practices:

> Best days of the week?
>
> Best time of the day?
>
> Best location?

When you think about creating the habit of finding space for yourself and your daily practices:

> What are some obstacles you have encountered?
>
> How have you managed life's disruptions?

When you think about yourself as your coach:

> What are the messages you are delivering to yourself?
>
> Have you discovered any sources of inspiration along the way?

Sometimes the bravest
and most important
thing you can do is
just show up.

BRENÉ BROWN

Beginning Enter your fitness space.

Silence your notifications.

Select music to accompany you today.

Movement Air Sharpie:

Imagine there is a sharpie on the center of your chin...

» Draw a square with that sharpie clockwise then counterclockwise.

Take 3 breaths.

Sit-Stand:

» Inhale to stand, exhale to sit.
» Complete 8-10 sit-stand repetitions.

Push-Ups:

» Place your hands on a desk, a wall, a counter or a sturdy table.
» Complete 4-6 push-ups.

Place your palm on your navel.

» Feel your belly rise as you inhale, lower as you exhale.
» Repeat 2 more times.

Mindset Finish the phrase:

» The best thing about my journey so far is...

Closing Reconnect and continue your day.

Connect

Most people know
their way around
the streets of
their hometown
better than they know
the anatomy of
their own body.

JILL MILLER

Then – Now

Historically, men always have had access to sports and physical activities.

But the concept of fitness for women is about 120 years old. Women were not encouraged to be physically active as it was thought to be harmful to their wellbeing.

Eventually, when society permitted, women began to explore a variety of options: calisthenics, VibroSlim, hula hoops, Pilates, yoga, aerobics, Jazzercize, Jane Fonda, Zumba, HIIT, CrossFit and so much more!

> There are many excellent websites, well-written and illustrated — simply Google the history of women and fitness.

> Better yet, dig in to see what fitness looked like the year you were born!

Fitness is ever-changing and predictable; some trends hold strong and true while others have a short shelf life.

Throughout your lifetime, you have observed and maybe even dabbled in some trends.

Trending...

Make a list of any recent fitness trends that have captured your attention?

What are they?

Maybe more interestingly, do you know anyone who has tried a recent fitness trend?

What was their review?

If you could go back in time:

Is there some fitness trend or innovation you wish you had access to right now?

If so, why does it appeal to you?

Beginning — What is the most nourishing, non-food related, something you can do for yourself today?

» Make a list of possibilities.

Select one something for yourself today.

Movement — Then, shift the idea into action.

» Go do that one something for yourself.

Mindset — Now, make some notes:

» Where did you go?

» Why was this something so good for you?

» How did you feel afterwards?

Closing — New concept to be used often:

Nourishment Day!

This kind of nourishment has so many layers:
so many ways to energize
your mind, body and energy —
it makes you an innovator!

My idea of exercise
is a good brisk sit.

Wonder

Having a sense of wonder tends to evaporate with age.

Problems need solutions.

Plans need actions.

Responsibilities need accountabilities.

It is interesting to see what happens when you sprinkle a bit of curiosity into the thought process.

The tone is different.

Less prescriptive.

Refreshed.

More optimistic.

Changing your language patterns creates space to discover the potential between *should* and *could!*

A sprinkle...

At any moment on any day, you are the only one who knows what is reasonable when it comes to fitting fitness into your day.

Instead of surrendering to the possibility of doing nothing at all, shift your language.

Your negotiations might become more energizing when you think of the possibilities.

Practice sprinkling some curiosity into these scenarios:

Instead of thinking, "I should go for a walk, but..."

Shift your mindset to becoming curious:

How could I move my body for the next 10 minutes?

Instead of thinking, "I shouldn't eat this."

Shift your mindset to becoming curious:

What would be a reasonable taste of this craving right now?

Practice sprinkling some curiosity into any fitness or wellness habit you are wrestling with:

Instead of thinking...

How could I...

Beginning

Curious...

» Where do you want your fitness studio to be today — move into that space.

» How can you create a space free from distractions — create that space.

MOVEMENT

What would you like to start your session with:

» Breathing?

» Sit-Stand?

» Push-Ups?

» Air Sharpies?

» Something else?

Start where you are.

Sequence the rest of this session as you decide.

Mindset

Curious...

» What did you do?

» How do you feel?

» Did you document this experience?

Closing

Reconnect.

Stay curious for the rest of today!

*If knowledge is power
then curiosity is
the muscle.*

DANIELLE LaPorte

Who

There are hundreds of reasons why women make a decision to get fit.

These reasons may be as simple as wanting to look good for an upcoming event, such as a reunion.

Or as serious as a life-or-death health situation.

The demand to dramatically alter one's lifestyle is often driven by one or two forces:

> A choice.

> Or a requirement.

Sometimes the *why* or the *what* reasons overshadow the *who*.

Truthfully...

Women often find themselves in the position of caregiver at various times in their lives.

Many of these same women look after others to the point they have little time or energy left for themselves.

So...

How will prioritizing YOUR fitness help you to help others when the need arises?

As you continue to push your fitness to the top of the day's priority list, consider:

How will changes to your fitness be beneficial to others you care for?

What would change?

Why is this of value to you?

Beginning

Enter your fitness space.

Sound check. Screens off.

Movement

Air Sharpie:

Imagine the shape of a triangle.

Draw two air triangles in two directions with:

» Your chin.

» Your dominant hand; your non-dominant hand.

» Your non-dominant arm; your dominant arm.

» Your right knee; your left knee.

» Your left heel; your right heel.

Movement Circuit Exercises:

» Sit-Stand: inhale to stand; exhale to sit.

» Push-Up: inhale to bend elbows; exhale to straighten.

» Balance on one foot: inhale, then exhale; repeat with the other foot.

Practice this circuit in the order listed.

» One breath for each repetition.

» Repeat the circuit 3-5 more times.

Closing

Carry on with your day as planned.

A simple reminder:
take care of
your wellbeing first,
everything after.

As you grow older,
you will discover
you have two hands.
One for helping
yourself; the other
for helping others.

MAYA ANGELOU

Her-story

Have you noticed whenever you see a medical professional and complete a health questionnaire, the questions are designed to determine your overall health based on your injuries, issues or illness history?

These questionnaires serve a valuable purpose: to assist your medical professional in supporting your well-being.

But have you also noticed these questionnaires remind you of personal details and information you may have forgotten?

Hopefully, your journey so far has also reminded you:

>Of your strengths.

>Of your abilities.

>Of your capacity to adapt and change.

Strength questionnaire...

Date:

You define strength as...

Name one of your strengths someone else has noticed...

Name one of your strengths few people know about...

Name the strongest, healthiest part of you...

When you think of your physical abilities, what is something you do well...

If you could use only one word, what word would describe you on your best day...

Name one strength you admire in others...

Beginning

Move into a fitness space that aligns best with your energy today.

Think about your energy.

Select a number of reps (between 4-10) that best align with you at this moment in time.

Movement

Sit-Stand: your reps.

Push-Up: your reps.

Balance:

» Stand tall and lift one foot off the floor.

» Hold for your rep count.

» Repeat on the other side.

Spine + Breath:

» Sit or stand then round your spine like a cat arches its back; reverse the spine and lift your heart upwards.

» In yoga, this pose is called Cat-Cow.

» Try it a couple more times to nourish your spine.

Mindset

Move to a resting position and put your feet up on the seat of a chair or against a wall.

» Think of some of your other strengths as you take 5 breaths.

Closing

When your feet touch back down, carry on with your strength-infused day.

Strong!

A river cuts through rock not because of its power but because of its persistence.

UNKNOWN

Your Manual

Fitness is best designed on a foundation of understandings related your physical form: past and present.

To generically set up or launch a fitness plan without considering your body is futile — which is why many such plans fizzle rather than sizzle.

The human body has a basic owner's manual - often found with varying degrees of detail under the heading of anatomy or human biology.

All humans would benefit from learning about basic joints and muscles of the body, as well as how they function.

You have one body.

Acquiring this language will be beneficial in so many ways.

R-e-s-p-e-c-t

Have you ever noticed how negatively people talk about their body parts?

So critical. So negative.

How about changing the slanguage into the language of the human body: anatomy!

See if you can convert the following:

Slang	Anatomical Term
butt	
muffin top	
bat wings	
schnozz	
spare tire	
the girls	
thunder thighs	
pot belly	

Let's give your body some credit by finishing the phrases below with respectable, anatomical language:

I love my...

I'm grateful for my...

Fitness Practice ♡ Practice Fitness

Beginning	What is the one thing you could do today that would benefit as many anatomical parts of you as possible?
	Keep your ideas in perspective:
	» How much time do you have?
	» What is your energy level today?
	» How will this nourish your mind and your body?
Movement	Just do it!
Mindset	Record what you did:
	» Make note of the anatomical parts that were nourished.
	» Any additional ideas you could try in the future?
Closing	Finish the phrase:
	» I am ...
	Carry on with your day.

The human body is amazing.
Your body is amazing

Get to know
your body better -
it'll be with you for
your entire lifetime!

UNKNOWN

Call to Action

You now have a refreshed understanding of your fitness history as well as personal preferences that align with who you are and how you live.

You have been practicing:

Setting and keeping fitness appointments.

Mindful breathing.

Strengthening your lower body.

Strengthening your upper body.

You have been *verb-ing*.

Not watching others.

Not reading about others.

Not thinking about the concept of fitness.

Doing!

Now we build on your practice by considering additional ingredients to keep you interested.

Fitness refreshment...

Think of all the ways you move your body on any given day.

From the moment you wake up.

Until the time you go to sleep.

Now, shift from thinking to documenting:

Make a list of all the ways, big or small, you have moved in the last 24 hours:

Then, flip back to your thoughts on page 45.

How have your movements changed?

Think of some new possibilities.

What are some new or modified verb-ing components you might consider adding to your fitness practices or daily movement patterns?

Injecting small amounts of novelty is refreshing!

Fitness Practice ♡ Practice Fitness

Beginning Move into your fitness space. Temporarily turn off all notifications.

Movement Breath Work: 3-6 repetitions

» Move your spine in and out of Cat-Cow, inhaling one direction; exhaling the other direction.

Breath Work + Arms: 3-6 repetitions

» Move your arms in a variety of directions as you inhale and exhale.

Breath Work + Sit-Stand: 3-6 repetitions

» Inhale and exhale as you transition from your feet to your seat

Breath Work + Push-ups: 3-6 repetitions

» Inhale and exhale as you bend then straighten your elbows.

Breath Work + Squats + Balance: 2-6 repetitions

» Stand in front of a seat of your choice. Lift one foot and balance for a moment then set it back down.

» Lower to your seat, pause to hover for a moment then sit.

Breath Work + Air Sharpie: 1-2 minutes

» Pick a geometric shape.

» Select parts of your body to move slowly in two directions

Closing Carry on with the rest of your day!

This is how
change happens:
one gesture,
one person,
one moment at a time.

KATY BOWMAN

Unfollow

This is an amazing time with unlimited access to innumerable sources of information and inspiration.

All you need to do is:

Connect with one or more of your social channels.

Like, subscribe and follow what interests you.

Before you know it, you'll be spending countless hours:

Watching.

Liking.

Following.

Then linking to similar sites for even more hours of sitting, watching, liking and following even more!

Precious minutes and hours of screen time pass with you in the audience.

Viewing.

Sometimes learning.

Most times just watching.

Is it time to change the channel?

Alternative channel...

Since beginning this journey:

How have your social media habits changed?

Here's your challenge:

Select two days this week to schedule a technology fast.

> No signing on.
> No watching.
> No liking.
> No following.
> No messaging.

To fill this screen time void, let's convert the next fitness practice into:

> Your fitness adventure!
> For your own, private social media channel!

Fitness Practice ♡ Practice Fitness

Beginning

Instead of watching someone else *do* fitness,
why not design a fitness adventure of your own?

Movement

Find a place to move your body and nourish your mind
without technology.

Then, document your fitness practice:

» Where did you go?
» What did you do?
» How did you *like* this moment in time?

If you were to do this again, what would you change?

Mindset

This practice invited you to be an influencer.

Your design was for your body, but it might be valuable
for others as well.

You are still on a technology fast so share what you
designed ONLY with those you care about, using a
method that doesn't require data or the Internet!

Closing

Carry on, influencing the rest of your day.

Your time is precious.
Optimize it!

In the most connected
time in history,
we're quickly losing
touch with ourselves.

RYDER CARROLL

Some thing

You are having one of *those* days:

> Your sense of time feels constricted.
>
> Your optimism fades with each passing hour.
>
> Your plans for today take on a life of their own.
>
> Your fitness practice seems unlikely.

Days like these happen. More often than we would like, but they are integral to life.

To recognize and adapt is the best strategy.

Many opt for the couch or table or some reclined position — often with food and beverages that make stress disappear momentarily, only to resurface with a new layer of stress, guilt or disappointment for not moving!

On these days, the mantra is simple:

> Something is better than nothing.

Having an express workout ready turns doing nothing into doing something!

Your time...

Woven somewhere in the mythology of fitness is the belief fitness takes an enormous amount of time: every day, every week, all year long.

For some, it does.

For most, it fits into the time available on any given day.

There may not be an enormous amount of time but, even on the busiest of days, there is still some time.

Take a few moments to simply consider:

If you had 3 minutes, what could you do for your fitness practice?

If you had 5 minutes, what could you do for your fitness practice?

If you had 7 minutes, what could you do for your fitness practice?

You can see how the thought process shifts:

From ◦ I don't have time for fitness today.

To ◦ This is the time I have for my fitness today.

Beginning Customize your space by clearing the clutter: space-wise or mind-wise.

Set your timer for 10 minutes, just for yourself.

Reminder: even on the busiest of days, you can find 10 minutes!

Movement Think — what could you do for:

» Your breath work?
» Your feet and legs?
» Your hands and arms?
» Your spine?
» Your breath again?
» Your energy?

Mindset When your 10 minutes are up, take a few extra moments to record what you did.

Closing Name it.

Save it.

Remember where it is.

*Use it whenever you have
one of those days!*

Time is free,
but it's priceless.
You can't own it,
but you can use it.
You can't keep it,
but you can spend it.
Once you've lost it,
you can never
get it back.

HARVEY MACKAY

Say It Isn't Solo

There are times when you want to team up with someone.

> A person to keep you company, to ensure you do what you set out to do and maybe share the experience with.

Having a friend or a partner be part of your fitness plan may be a desired element of your fitness, but truthfully, you will be the one stepping into most of your sessions on your own.

Your schedule, your energy and your body will have completely different needs than anyone else.

Over time, you will find it easier to integrate your fitness into your life.

> Being solo will simplify things.

You will fit fitness into your day when it works for you and your day.

> If you meet others on the journey, that is a bonus.

Your own company...

Going solo doesn't mean being silent or lonely or serious.

What audio companions inspire you:

If you were to join a group-based fitness class or club:

How can you be with others in a complimentary rather than competitive or comparative way?

Trying new things or places can be intimidating if you are flying solo.

What are some considerations for:

Your personal safety?

You confidently arriving on time to a fitness space of your choosing?

Anything else of importance to you?

Beginning

Define your fitness space.
Settle in and create a flow with your breath and your arms.

Movement

Design your practice with the following invitations:

» Move for 2 minutes.

» Spine Work: Cat-Cow, 2-4 breaths.

» Push-Up: 8-10 times.

» Move for 2 minutes.

» Air Sharpie: pick a shape then move your chin, arms, hips, knees, heels.

» Sit-Squat: 8-10 times.

» Move for 2 minutes.

» Balance: stand on one foot; then the other.

» Take 6 energizing breaths.

» Breath Work + Spine Movement: 2-4 breaths.

Mindset

Next time, invite someone to do this fitness practice with you — select a different day, time and place.

Then, ask that same someone to invite you into their fitness space.

What a great way to share and enjoy each other's company!

Closing

Your fitness practice is accessible wherever you are. On your own or with others.

Your body. Your strength.
Your options. Your practice.

When women take care
of their health,
they become
their best friend.

MAYA ANGELOU

They Say

They...

    Are a noisy and opinionated bunch!

They...

    Have opinions, ideas and innovations, as well as services and products for sale.

They...

    Often say things that have the most relevance when you are at your lowest energy.

Their premise...

    If you do this, that will happen.

Your response...

    You sign up and pay up.

Sometimes what they say is exactly what you need.

    Other times, it's a distraction.

Most often, you simply need to access your...

    THEY SAY filter!

You say...

They say...	What if...	You say...
Exercise first thing in the morning.	You work first thing in the morning or your job is shift work?	
Prioritize your fitness.	Your young children or elder parents are a priority?	
Weekly massages are essential.	You don't have health benefits.	
Walk 10,000 steps per day.	You have issues with your feet.	
Exercise 6 days per week.	You travel for work or for pleasure?	
You should only eat organic.	You are living on a tight budget.	
Maybe something else..	Your reality...	You say...

Beginning

You are the coach today.
Take a moment before beginning your session to check in:

» How did you sleep last night?
» How much time did you sit, stand, lift or move today?
» How much time did you have to hydrate, nourish and digest?
» How much energy is required for the balance of your day?

Movement

With this in mind, move into your practice space.

Focus on one element of this practice at a time; selecting the movement, the duration and the intensity.

What will you do for your:

» Breath Work:
» Spine Work:
» Arm Work:
» Leg Work:
» Balance:
» Anything else:

Mindset

You are becoming an expert with regard to better understanding your own body and the fitness elements that feel good.

Closing

If you were to join the *they say* choir, what would you add to this conversation?

Empowered.

What people say,
what people do,
and what people say
they do are entirely
different things.

Reflection

When you look at the journey thus far, have you noticed a pattern of consistency — spaces that work well for you and your fitness practices:

> Best days of the week?
>
> Best time of the day?
>
> Best location?

When you think about creating the habit of finding space for yourself and your daily practices:

> What are some obstacles you have encountered?
>
> How have you managed life's disruptions?

When you think about yourself as your coach:

> What are the messages you are delivering to yourself?
>
> Have you discovered any sources of inspiration along the way?

Sometimes you will never know the value of a moment until it becomes a memory.

DR. SEUSS

Beginning

Move into your fitness space.

Sound check. Distraction check. Energy check.

Movement

Paint the Globe: 1-2 minutes

» Imagine you are standing inside a glass snow globe.

» Without moving your feet, imagine painting the inside of this globe with your palms — above, beside, under and behind where you are standing.

Sit-Stand + Challenge: 10-12 reps

» Try a variety of seats.

Push-Up + Challenge: 4-6 reps

» Lift one leg, push-up, lower the leg.

» Then repeat with the other leg.

Balance + Challenge: 1-3 breaths

» Lift one foot off the floor, gaze right then left. Repeat on the other side.

Repeat this circuit 2-3 more times.

Mindset

Your practices can be as long or as short, as relaxing or as intense as you decide. Every day.

Closing

Find a nourishing way to celebrate your journey thus far sometime today.

Carpe diem!

Continue

Watch your habits,
for they become
your posture.

Watch your posture,
for it creates boundaries.

Watch your boundaries,
for they restrict
your growth.

Watch your restrictions,
for they create immobility.

Watch your immobility,
for it becomes
your illness.

KATY BOWMAN

Calendar Dates

Have you ever experienced that day…the one where you promise yourself something is going to change, in this case, your commitment to fitness?

So committed are you to the process of fitness, you have a plan to radically change your world.

It's well thought-out.

Detailed.

Fail-proof.

And then, your day starts with something you forgot or didn't anticipate: all components of your plan to practice fitness evaporate.

All plans to become fit need to actually fit into life.

Many use a system to keep track of schedules, appointments and commitments.

Within this reality is an understanding:

All things are subject to change.

This is a great space to pause to look at how you plan your life and your commitment to fitness.

More experts...

When it comes to time management...THEY are also a noisy bunch!

They say you should use:

- Your phone or your tablet.
- Google Calendar or Outlook.
- Day timer or bullet journal.
- Paper only or technology only.
- And the list goes on and on!

It might be beneficial to shift from listening to the experts to asking yourself a few essential questions:

How do you record an important future date in such a way you won't forget it and, most importantly, remember to not book something else at this time?

Does your system really work most of the time?

How can it improve?

What do you need to set-up, or revise, a reliable system so it can be used on a yearly, monthly, weekly and daily basis?

How will your fitness practice appointments be scheduled alongside life's other priorities?

Beginning

Move into your fitness space.

Consider:

» How much time do you have for this session?

» What is your energy level?

Movement

Go back through your notes and select a fitness practice from your past.

Review the sequence.

Now, shuffle the details...

Mix the order in such a way it looks like the perfect session for you today.

Coach yourself through your refreshed practice.

Mindset

Take a moment:

» Is this a design worth documenting?

» If so, record your refreshed plan.

If not, remember, you can mix the order of your fitness practices so long as you take time to check in with yourself before you start and after you finish the session.

Closing

Take a long breath to conclude today's session, then carry on with your day.

The simplest change can be the most refreshing!

Have regular hours for
work and play;
make each day
both useful
and pleasant,
and prove that you
understand the worth
of time by
enjoying it well.

LOUISA MAY ALCOTT

Ceremony

Depending on how you plan or coordinate your fitness sessions, there is more to the process than just showing up and just doing it.

It's kind of like thinking about this time for yourself as being either fast food or fine dining.

> Fast food often leaves little time to savor or appreciate anything other than the convenience.

> Fine dining invites all the senses to the table so the experience is much more than eating.

When you come to this time of the day, your fitness practice, take a few moments to set your table.

Because this is your time, your choice, your fitness ceremony.

Fitness pairings...

Who says fitness practices must always be practices?

Why can't fitness be paired seamlessly with other things you like to do?

For example, instead of:

Meeting a friend for a coffee...

>   Meet a friend, then walk for a coffee.

Sitting and watching TV at the end of the day...

>   Set your timer to pause the program every 20 minutes to take a movement break.

Taking young child to a playground...

>   Try some of the playground equipment yourself!

When you think of your life and your movement patterns, what are some other pairings you could consider:

In your own company or in the company of others?

Beginning   What if you infused today's practice with your imagination?

Movement   Some possibilities...

Select a light object, pick it up and set it down using the strength of your legs.

Clear a space and use your imagination to move your body as if you are swimming, skiing, skating, skipping or walking along a ledge.

Set your timer, move in one or more of these patterns.

Pick a favorite song, one that invites you to move.

Play the song and dance like no one is watching.

Mindset   Make a note of what you did or any other ideas that came to mind.

Fitness practice ceremonies have infinite possibilities!

Closing   Carry on with your day.

Imagine!

*Exercising should not
be a task, a chore,
a punishment or
a coping mechanism.
It should be liberating,
energizing and
empowering.*

ERWAN LE CORRE

Your Vows

The longest relationship you will have with any body is your relationship with your body:

> You will live your entire life together, in sickness, in health and everything in between.

For the most part, your body does what it needs to do — keeping you alive: breathing, sleeping, digesting, eliminating.

This body of yours is most forgiving when you:

> Get less sleep than required.
>
> Eat less nourishing food than desired.
>
> Recover from bumps, bruises and illness.
>
> Worry about things that may never happen.

Like a valued piece of property, wear and tear can be preserved or reversed with a little restoration.

> Making this an opportune time to renew your fitness vows!

Fitness vows...

Go back to page 71 and reread who you were getting fit for.

Think about you at this point in the journey...

What has changed?

Why is continuing to practice fitness a priority?

How can you deepen your commitment to feeling fit?

After rereading, reflecting and reconnecting:

Write your fitness vows:

From this day forward...

Beginning

Move into your fitness space.

Settle into a resting position.

Elevate your feet, support your head and your spine.

Relax.

Mindset

Think about all the incredibly amazing things your body is doing for your wellbeing right now.

Review your refreshed fitness vows as you close your eyes.

In this space of stillness, let your renewed vows settle into your very being.

Stay in this space for as long as your day permits.

Closing

When your feet touch down, carry on with a sense of renewal!

Recommitted to your fitness!

*I believe the body has
its own intelligence,
an inner memory
of what it is
to be right.*

YAMUNA ZAKE

Arrived

You, day by day, as your life permitted, have set aside time to practice fitness.

By doing so, you are more aware of:

The importance of breathing.

The value of strength in your body.

Increasing your sense of balance and mobility.

Some of you may have added other fitness components or continued with fitness routines that were already in place.

You understand the importance of making time for your personal fitness, however long or short.

Done well, fitness gives you the energy to do what you *want* to do as well as what you *need* to do.

Ultimately, looking after your physical wellbeing comes first...so you can take care of everything else.

This may be a journey you repeat and refine, but for now, it's important to acknowledge:

You are here!

You know yourself...

At the beginning of this journey:

Getting started was a focus.

So was finding an accessible space for your fitness practice.

Now that you are at the end of this journey, it's important to reset your GPS:

Where are you going?

How do you think you want to get there?

All endings have new beginnings, enriched with life's experiences:

What have you learned that will keep you on this path of your design and your choosing?

Reflection

When you look at the journey thus far, have you noticed a pattern of consistency — spaces that work well for you and your fitness practices:

> Best days of the week?
>
> Best time of the day?
>
> Best location?

When you think about creating the habit of finding space for yourself and your daily practices:

> What are some obstacles you have encountered?
>
> How have you managed life's disruptions?

When you think about yourself as your coach:

> What are the messages you are delivering to yourself?
>
> Have you discovered any sources of inspiration along the way?

*She believed
she could
so she did.*

Unknown

Beginning   Set up your fitness space for today.

Movement   Breath Work: 5-10 breaths.

Paint the Globe: 2 minutes.

Balance: 4-6 times.

   Walk the edge of an imaginary line on the floor or a yoga mat.

   Then walk that same line backwards.

Imagery: 6 steps

   Take steps over an imaginary object.

   Then take steps ducking under an imaginary object.

Push-Up: 6-10 reps.

   Your choice.

Sit-Stand: 6-10 reps.

   Your choice.

Spine Work: 3-6 breaths.

   Cat-Cow.

Mindset   Every so often, injecting a bit of novelty can inject new energy into any daily practice.

Closing   You have arrived.

Success!

A Fork in the Road

This journey was not about running a marathon...

But it's great if you did.

It was not about losing a set amount of body weight...

But it's great if you did.

It was not about fitting into a certain clothing size..

But it's great if you did.

It was not about purchasing apparel...

But it's great if you did.

It was not about purchasing equipment...

Instead, you used a space, wall, floor and chair.

And here you are!

There was no mention of cardio, conditioning, calories, carbs or competition.

The only comparisons were you reflecting on your changes.

This journey was about:

    Less watching, more practicing.

    Less being influenced, more self-influencing.

    Less knowing, more learning.

Your daily fitness habit may still be evolving, but it is no longer elusive.

The key to this evolution is setting aside time and space for your fitness practice every single day.

As time progresses and you age alongside time, your fitness practice will need revisions based on how your body feels and what it needs to feel fit in real time.

The more you know about yourself, the more open you will be to continue to learn.

    As you know, there is no shortage of information. The priority is to filter, then select what will work for you.

Simply, fitness is a feeling that leads to:

    Contentment in your skin.

    Contentment in your movements.

    Contentment in your life.

Beginning

Move into your fitness space.

Go back through your notes and select a fitness practice.

Repeat the practice, making any changes necessary for today.

Mindset

Time to consider your next fitness steps.

> How do you want to feel when you arrive at the next fork in the road?

Take a moment to be grateful for :

> Your efforts.
> Your commitment.
> Your amazing-ness.

Prepare

To relaunch.

You know what to do!

Practice fitness, some way, some form, some time, every single day.

*It is not happiness that
makes us grateful.*

*It is gratitude that
makes us happy!*

Your Resources

You have been encouraged to unfollow, but keep learning.

In essence, to shift from watching to engaging; from following to leading; from sitting to moving; from listening to creating.

If you haven't already done so, you may want to build a resource library of your own. A library that fortifies your knowledge and amplifies the daily habit of fitness.

> Some of you might build a physical library with shelves, books, magazines or any other print material.

> Others will opt to have a virtual library with links, favorites, reading pages readily available for quick reference or updates.

Over time, you will read, listen and watch many wise mentors; continue curating a short list of your preferences.

Keep your resource list as current as your fitness practices.

My Favorites

I am always on the lookout for inspiration — it keeps my practice interesting and fresh.

That said, I do have four sources that remain consistent. Any book, link or post by these women is always on my radar:

Yamuna Zake

Jill Miller

Sage Rountree

Katy Bowman

If you don't have one already, start to look at acquiring an anatomy book. You will find quite an assortment of formats, from the detailed medical guides to simple overviews for children – any of which will enhance your understanding of your amazing human body.

Fitness trends are perennial: they are continually trending!

Fads can inject novelty into your practice as can anything tried and true.

Keep injecting the right amount of spice or sweetness to keep yourself engaged.

Stay open to all fitness possibilities.

Again

Practicing fitness, for the most part, is an individual journey.

There may be connections along the way, these are intersections — spaces where interests and personalities meet, but your actual fitness experience can only be felt by you, managed by you and redesigned by you.

Fitness is a feeling!

As life continues, so will the evolution of your fitness practice.

As your practice evolves, so will your understanding of YOU!

Don't you know that women are the only works of art?

DON HENLEY

Create

You know all those things you've always wanted to do?
You should do them!

ANONYMOUS

If, then, so

IF you have read a few pages a day; thought about fitness, opened your mind to fitness possibilities in your life, you are ready to put the practice in real time.

Day by day.

Week by week.

Month by month.

THEN you can consider what day of the week you will commit to sitting down and mapping out your commitments, including your fitness practice appointments:

SO, on the day you selected, map out your week in the following order:

Work or other daily commitments:
These are categorized as *non-negotiable*.

Social or other details:
These are *negotiable*.

Spaces for fitness practices:
These are *essential*.

Remember...focus on the step in front of you not the entire staircase.

UNKNOWN

Sample One Week Plan: Busy

Go back through this book and select a couple of fitness practice elements to weave into your weekly plan.

Here is a sample based on a busy week.

You decide the duration, the distance, the repetitions...

I: Monday & Thursday

Breath + Arm Circles
Cat–Cow
Air Sharpie

II: Tuesday & Friday

Breath + Cat–Cow
Chair Squats
Wall Push-ups

III: Saturday

Walk
Legs Up the Wall
Belly Breaths

IV: Sunday

Rest, relaxation, prepare for next week

Sample One Week Plan: Vacation

Go back through this book and select different fitness practice elements to weave into your weekly plan.

Here is a sample based on a vacation week.

You decide the duration, the distance, the repetitions...

I: Monday & Saturday: Travel days

Airplane Breath + Belly Breathing
Airport Sit-Hover-Stand
Airport Steps: walking while waiting

II: Tuesday, Wednesday & Friday

Before heading out for sightseeing:

Paint the Globe
Wall Push-ups
Wall Chair Squats

Before bed:

Air Sharpie

III: Sunday
Walk
Legs up the Wall
Prepare for next week

Fitness is

A journey.

One with infinite possibilities — all of which you can customize specifically for your needs, your energy and your time.

If you wish to continue the journey with me, watch for the second book in this collection; more creative ways to move your body with some fresh ingredients for your designs.

Until then, practice.

Smile.

Carry on.

Be fearless.
Know that all
will be provided
at the right time.

YOGI TEA AFFIRMATION

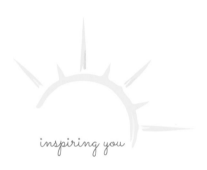

inspiring you

Heather has been on a similar fitness journey — she is not a celebrity trainer, a former dancer, a retired Olympian or any other extraordinary human being.

She is a fitness whisperer — to herself first and, then, to anyone interested in discovering the *contentment* personal fitness creates.

Manufactured by Amazon.ca
Bolton, ON

33750381R00079